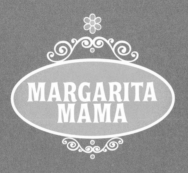

MARGARITA MAMA

Library of Congress Cataloging in Publication Number: 2007938202
ISBN: 978-1-59474-215-6
Printed in Singapore
Typeset in Helvetica Neue, Shag Expert

Designed by Bryn Ashburn
Illustrations by Lisa Henderling
Edited by Melissa Wagner

Distributed in North America by Chronicle Books
680 Second Street
San Francisco, CA 94107

10 9 8 7 6 5 4 3 2 1

Quirk Books
215 Church Street
Philadelphia, PA 19106
www.quirkbooks.com

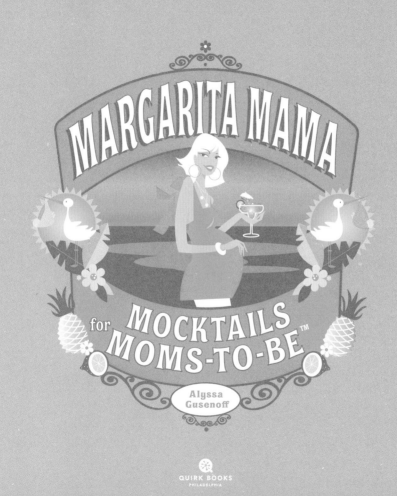

MARGARITA MAMA

MOCKTAILS for MOMS-TO-BE™

Alyssa
Gusenoff

QUIRK BOOKS
PHILADELPHIA

To
Dan and Zachary,
the only ingredients
I need!

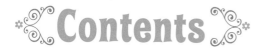

Contents

ON THE ROCKS

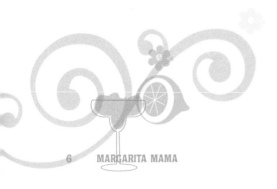

MARTINIS & MORE

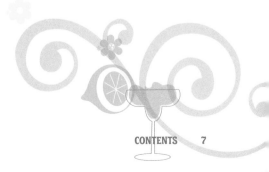

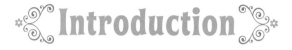 Introduction

I'll never forget that wonderful moment when the concept of the Margarita Mama was born.

I was newly pregnant. (Translation: No alcohol allowed!) It was a hot summer day. I was visiting my in-laws at their beach house, and all my summer-trained instincts called out for a real margarita. Everyone else was indulging in a chilly, sprightly, refreshing cocktail. Sure, none of *them* were pregnant—but what about meeeeee?

The bottled ice water I held in my hand just didn't cut it!

I walked inside. I looked up. And there it was: a blender, staring down at me tauntingly from the kitchen shelf. With sudden resolve, I tugged open the refrigerator and began pulling out ingredients. I started with some limeade. I added a dash of orange juice. I took a sip. I added some ginger ale and peach juice. I turned the blender on high. And there it was—perfect! The Margarita Mama was born.

I happily rimmed a glass with salt, poured in my creation, and headed outside to join the fun.

The Margarita Mama got me hooked. After that, I was determined to create non-alcoholic drinks that would quench the thirst of pregnant women like me during the long months ahead. I immediately went to the local grocery store and bought every type of juice, soda, frozen fruit, and mixer I could find.

As I stared at the kitchen table covered with ingredients, I began to get creative. Trial and error seemed to be the best strategy. At first many of the drinks were too sweet or too sour, but I soon began to find good nonalcoholic substitutes. Pineapple juice turned out to be a tasty stand-in for rum, and ginger ale makes an excellent tequila replacement.

When morning sickness set in, my husband assumed the role of the official taster. After dinner, we would line up the ingredients, and I would start mixing. When a drink received his seal of approval, I sampled the finished product.

My initial idea was to have just a few thirst-quenchers that I could easily mix for any occasion. But soon I began to think long-term. A new drink for every week of pregnancy, and then some! Creating these new drinks was something to look forward to besides stretch marks and fatigue.

After finalizing the recipes, I decided it was time to venture out of my kitchen. A good friend invited me over for a dinner party, so I packed up the ingredients for the Nothing Fits Fizz and was on my way. At the party I made myself a drink and offered it to another pregnant friend, and then others wanted a taste. Before I knew it, everyone was drinking the Nothing Fits Fizz while the bottle of pinot noir sat unopened on the counter. If these drinks hit the spot for some of my non-pregnant girlfriends, I knew they would be a hit with pregnant women as well.

As my pregnancy progressed, I read pregnancy books that opined about the benefits of a balanced diet full of fruits and vegetables. Yet as my cravings set in, I was more likely to reach for a bag of potato chips than a handful of fruit. My mocktails became my main source of fruit. I could sip a healthy, fruity beverage while I ate my chips. It was the best of both worlds!

I admit that the idea of a glass of wine was a nice light at the end of the tunnel when I entered my final trimester. However, I didn't long for a cocktail the way I longed for a margarita that summer day on the porch with my friends and family. In fact, I'm sure that next summer I will be sitting happily on my in-laws' porch sipping a Nothing Fits Fizz as I long to squeeze back into my pre-pregnancy jeans!

Cheers!

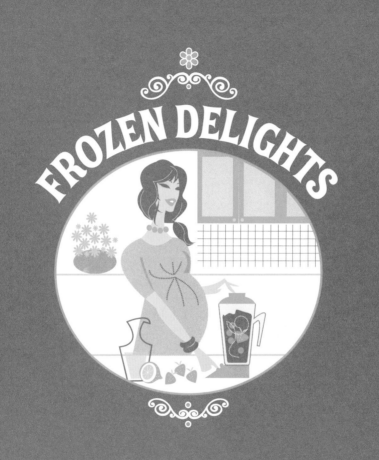

FROZEN DELIGHTS

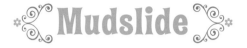

Mudslide

It's time to indulge! The Mudslide serves as a delicious drink as well as the perfect dessert—there's no better way to get the extra calcium and calories your pregnant body needs.

- **2 scoops coffee ice cream**
- **½ cup chocolate milk**
- **1 cup ice**
- **2 tablespoons chocolate syrup, divided**
- **Whipped cream, for garnish**

Place the coffee ice cream, chocolate milk, ice, and 1 tablespoon of chocolate syrup in a blender and blend on medium speed until creamy. As an extra treat, garnish with whipped cream and the rest of the chocolate syrup. Serve immediately.

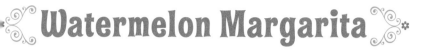

Watermelon Margarita

When every part of your body feels swollen, it's time to sit back with a Watermelon Margarita. The watermelon will relieve water retention, and the sweet taste will help you forget that your rings don't fit anymore.

- **1 cup frozen watermelon chunks**
- **5 ounces ginger ale**
- **1 tablespoon lime juice**
- **Watermelon slice, for garnish**

Place all the ingredients in a blender and blend on medium speed until the watermelon is pureed and smooth. Garnish with a fresh slice and enjoy immediately.

A Toast to Your Health!

Water retention, or bloat, is a common pregnancy problem. If you're looking to remedy the discomfort but want to avoid taking pills or chemical supplements, be aware that certain foods, including watermelons, act as natural diuretics. In addition to its bloat-reducing properties, watermelon is an excellent source of lycopene, vitamin C, beta carotene, and folic acid.

White Russian

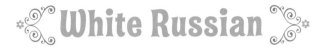

Fight the frustrations of travel restrictions with a White Russian, a world of yummy flavors that will take your mind to distant destinations.

- **1 cup vanilla ice cream or frozen yogurt**
- **½ cup ginger ale**
- **1 tablespoon coffee-flavored syrup**
- **2 tablespoons chocolate syrup, divided**
- **½ cup ice**

Place the vanilla ice cream/frozen yogurt, ginger ale, coffee-flavored syrup, 1 tablespoon chocolate syrup, and ice in a blender and blend on medium-high speed until smooth. Garnish with the remaining tablespoon of chocolate syrup and serve immediately.

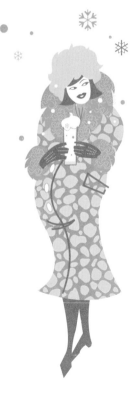

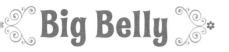

Big Belly

Round out your day with the Big Belly, a delicious source of potassium and calcium. One of the biggest benefits of pregnancy is the ability to hide a few ounces gained while partaking in culinary pleasures—so enjoy!

- 1 cup vanilla ice cream or frozen yogurt
- 1/2 banana
- 1 tablespoon maple syrup
- 1/4 cup pineapple juice
- 1/4 cup ice

Place all the ingredients in a blender and pulse on medium speed until the banana is pureed and all the ingredients are blended together. Serve immediately.

Bottoms Up!

What to wear? Fortunately, maternity clothes have become quite stylish and are widely available at all national chains. There's even maternity lingerie! But to avoid spending too much on outfits you'll wear only a short time, buy smart. Splurge on well-fitting pants and a dressy skirt but opt for less-expensive oversized tops to mix and match. And don't forget to ask friends who recently gave birth whether they have items to pass on. Recycling is the most economical alternative!

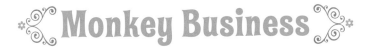

Monkey Business

After a long day of doctors' appointments and birthing classes, sometimes you just feel like monkeying around. Here's how.

- 1 frozen banana
- 1 scoop vanilla ice cream or frozen yogurt
- 1 scoop chocolate ice cream or frozen yogurt
- ½ cup ice
- 1 tablespoon chocolate syrup

Combine all the ingredients in a blender and pulse on medium speed until the banana is pureed and the ingredients are fully blended into a smooth, thick shake. Serve immediately.

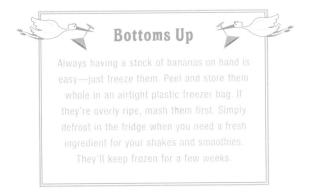

Bottoms Up

Always having a stock of bananas on hand is easy—just freeze them. Peel and store them whole in an airtight plastic freezer bag. If they're overly ripe, mash them first. Simply defrost in the fridge when you need a fresh ingredient for your shakes and smoothies. They'll keep frozen for a few weeks.

Baby Shower Shake

When all the girls gather to celebrate your baby's future "birthday," treat them to a wonderful Baby Shower Shake. Not only does it taste great, it also offers the nutritional benefits of blueberries, which are full of antioxidants and vitamin C.

- ¼ cup fresh or frozen blueberries (reserve 4 or 5 for garnish)
- ½ banana
- 1 scoop vanilla ice cream or frozen yogurt
- ¼ cup blueberry juice
- ¼ cup ice
- Whipped cream, for garnish

Place all the ingredients in a blender and blend at medium-high speed until fully combined into a nice, thick shake. Garnish with whipped cream and the reserved blueberries. Enjoy immediately.

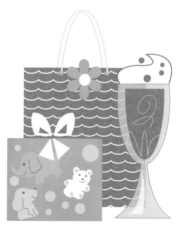

Strawberry Piña Colada

Soon you may find that your financial priorities change from splurging on an island vacation to purchasing a decked-out crib and glider. But you can always remember the taste of the tropics with a Strawberry Piña Colada.

- **4 to 5 fresh or frozen strawberries (reserve one for garnish)**
- **5 ounces pineapple juice**
- **2 tablespoons coconut cream**
- **1/2 cup ice**
- **Pineapple wedge, for garnish (optional)**

Place all the ingredients in a blender and blend until smooth. Garnish with a fresh strawberry and/or pineapple wedge and serve immediately.

Bottoms Up

Coconut cream is sold as either a liquid or a concentrated powder and is available in most grocery stores. In addition to its mildly sweet flavor, this versatile ingredient offers many nutritional benefits, including boosting metabolism and immune systems. Like coconut oil, coconut cream contains lauric acid, which is also found in breast milk and is considered to have antimicrobial properties. Use coconut cream as a substitute in recipes that call for milk; it's especially good in hot chocolate and smoothies.

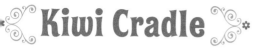 Kiwi Cradle

Having trouble putting together that new crib or bassinet? Put away your screwdriver and fix up a Kiwi Cradle instead. With just three easy ingredients and simple, straightforward instructions, this is one cradle you won't mind making again and again.

- 2 kiwis, peeled and cut into cubes (reserve 1 slice for garnish)
- 2 ounces lemonade
- 4 ounces lemon-lime soda

Puree the kiwi in a blender. Add the lemonade and lemon-lime soda. Blend until smooth. Serve immediately, garnished with a fresh kiwi slice.

A Toast to Your Health!

Kiwi is a great addition to a pregnant woman's diet, and not just for its tangy, refreshing taste. It's a great source of folate, a B vitamin that helps prevent neural birth defects such as anencephaly and spina bifida. For pregnant women, doctors recommend a daily intake of 800 micrograms of folate or folic acid, folate's synthetic equivalent and a common ingredient in prenatal vitamins. The additional 90 micrograms supplied in the Kiwi Cradle are a great excuse to indulge in this drink anytime.

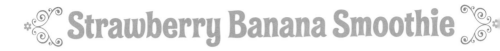

Strawberry Banana Smoothie

When you're too tired to eat, it can seem impossible to get five servings of fruit a day. The Strawberry Banana Smoothie is refreshing and gives you more than half the recommended fruit servings you need for the day—giving you more time to rest!

- **4 to 5 frozen strawberries (reserve one for garnish)**
- **1 frozen banana**
- **½ cup strawberry yogurt**
- **½ cup milk**

Place all the ingredients in a blender and blend on medium-high speed until smooth and creamy. Garnish with a strawberry and serve immediately.

Frozen Root Beer Float

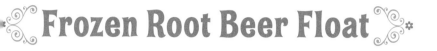

You're never too old for a Frozen Root Beer Float! Consider doubling the recipe—your husband is sure to demand a taste when he spies this frosty treat.

- **4 ounces root beer**
- **2 scoops vanilla ice cream or frozen yogurt**

Place all the ingredients in a blender and blend on medium speed until fully incorporated into a nice, thick shake. Grab a straw and enjoy immediately.

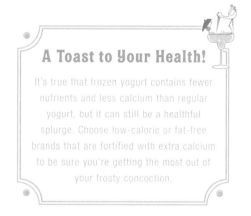

A Toast to Your Health!

It's true that frozen yogurt contains fewer nutrients and less calcium than regular yogurt, but it can still be a healthful splurge. Choose low-calorie or fat-free brands that are fortified with extra calcium to be sure you're getting the most out of your frosty concoction.

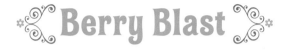

Berry Blast

The Berry Blast is a frozen delight that's perfect for sharing, so invite all your friends over for a "berry" good time! Who can resist such naturally sweet, good-for-you ingredients?

- ¼ **cup frozen blueberries**
- ¼ **cup frozen raspberries**
- **2 to 3 frozen strawberries**
- ¼ **cup vanilla yogurt**
- ½ **banana**
- ½ **cup milk**
- **1 fresh strawberry, for garnish**

Place all the ingredients in a blender and pulse until the fruit is pureed and the ingredients are fully blended. Garnish with a fresh strawberry and serve immediately.

A Toast to Your Health!

Berries offer many diverse health benefits, packing a punch of vitamins, phytochemicals (which help prevent diseases), and lutein (for improved vision). Consider adding these naturally sweet treats to your diet. One fun way to do so is to organize a pick-your-own outing at a local farm. Nothing compares to freshly gathered pints of delicious berries, but if it's not the season, frozen berries will do in a pinch.

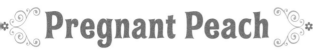

Pregnant Peach

Next time you find yourself reaching for a not-so-healthy candy bar, try a Pregnant Peach instead. The combination of peaches and lemonade will provide your body with extra vitamin C and leave you feeling energized and refreshed—naturally!

- ½ cup ice
- ½ cup frozen peach slices (reserve a few for garnish)
- 6 ounces lemonade
- 4 ounces iced tea
- 2 ounces peach juice

Place all the ingredients in a blender and pulse on medium speed just until smooth. Garnish with a few peach slices and serve immediately.

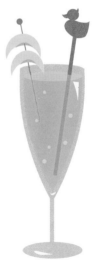

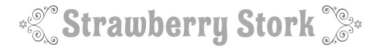

Strawberry Stork

Now that you've learned about the birds and the bees, it's time to familiarize yourself with the Strawberry Stork, ready to deliver refreshment anytime of the day or night.

- **6 to 7 frozen strawberries (reserve one for garnish)**
- **6 ounces lemon-lime soda**

Place all the ingredients in a blender and pulse on medium-high speed just until smooth. Garnish with a fresh strawberry.

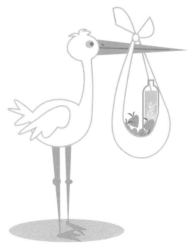

Zachary Daiquiri

With its tangy flavor of peach and mango, the Zachary Daiquiri—named after my newborn!—is sure to deliver satisfaction both before and after your own little one arrives.

- 3 to 4 frozen peach slices
- 4 to 5 frozen mango chunks
- 6 ounces ginger ale
- 1 ounce fresh orange juice
- 1 fresh peach slice (for garnish)

Place all the ingredients in a blender and blend on medium-high speed until smooth. Serve immediately, garnished with a fresh peach slice.

A Toast to Your Health!

A popular tropical fruit native to southern and Southeast Asia, the mango is a good source of vitamins A and C as well as beta carotene, a nutrient that's important for a baby's vision and immune system. Its sweet, unique taste can be used to enhance traditional dishes such as salsa and chutney, not to mention livening up a bowl of bland (but healthful!) high-protein cereal.

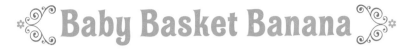

Baby Basket Banana

Enjoy the ease of food shopping now . . . once the little one arrives, routine errands will become day-long affairs. Throw some fruit into your basket and check out the Baby Basket Banana.

- ½ banana
- ¼ cup frozen blueberries
- 3 to 4 frozen or fresh peach slices
- 1 ounce orange juice
- 4 ounces ginger ale

Place all the ingredients in a blender and pulse on medium-high speed until all the fruit is pureed and the drink has a smooth, frothy consistency. Serve immediately.

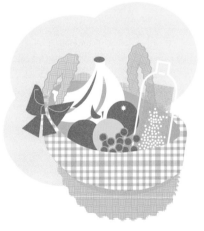

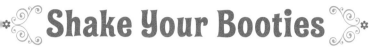

Shake Your Booties

Here's a rich, creamy drink that will give you enough energy to dance the night away.

- ¼ cup frozen or fresh blueberries (reserve 4 to 5 for garnish)
- 2 tablespoons coconut cream
- 1 scoop vanilla ice cream or frozen yogurt
- 1 cup ice
- Whipped cream, for garnish

Place all the ingredients in a blender and blend on medium-high speed until creamy. Garnish with whipped cream and top with a few blueberries.

Bottoms Up!

Myths abound about what pregnant women should and should not do. Although in the past, exercise was frowned upon, today women are encouraged to be active during pregnancy. One of the best ways to stay fit, relieve stress, build muscle, and strengthen your heart is through dancing. Consider a low-impact style, such as belly dancing. Just be sure to discuss your new exercise plans with your doctor and adjust your regime as needed throughout your pregnancy.

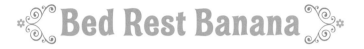

Bed Rest Banana

Sit back, put your feet up, and sip a tropical-inspired libation that is sure to please, especially when you're not allowed to get out of bed for a few weeks.

- **1 banana**
- **1/3 cup pineapple juice**
- **1/2 cup seltzer**
- **1/4 cup ice**
- **Fresh pineapple slice, for garnish**

Place all the ingredients in a blender and pulse on medium speed until the banana and ice are combined and smooth. Garnish with a fresh pineapple slice and enjoy immediately.

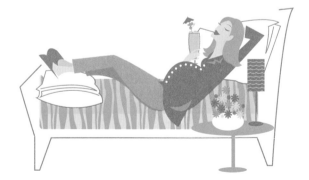

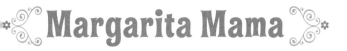

Margarita Mama

This nonalcoholic version of the Tex-Mex classic will have you wishing for a bowl of chips and salsa! This recipe makes enough for six people, so recruit your teetotaling friends and enjoy a pitcher together. If you're feeling extra generous, share some with your alcohol-drinking buddies, too.

- Kosher salt
- 12 ounces frozen limeade
- 6 ounces orange juice
- 10 ounces water
- 2 ounces peach juice
- 8 ounces ginger ale
- 1 cup ice
- 6 lime wedges

Pour the kosher salt on a plate, rub the rim of each of six glasses with a lime wedge, and dip the rims to coat with salt. Pour the limeade, orange juice, water, peach juice, ginger ale, and ice into a blender and blend until smooth. Serve in the salted margarita glasses, garnished with a lime wedge. Makes 6 servings.

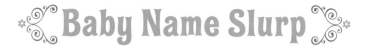

Baby Name Slurp

While you're poring over dozens of books, agonizing over what to name your baby, savor this relaxing blend of flavors. They'll help you put all those choices into perspective.

- **1 cup frozen or fresh mango**
- **4 to 5 frozen or fresh strawberries (reserve one for garnish)**
- **5 ounces lemon-lime soda**
- **1 ounce ginger ale**

Place all the ingredients in a blender and pulse on medium speed until the fruit is pureed and smooth. Garnish with a strawberry and serve immediately.

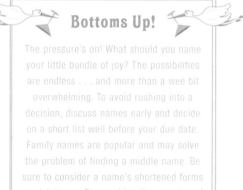

Bottoms Up!

The pressure's on! What should you name your little bundle of joy? The possibilities are endless . . . and more than a wee bit overwhelming. To avoid rushing into a decision, discuss names early and decide on a short list well before your due date. Family names are popular and may solve the problem of finding a middle name. Be sure to consider a name's shortened forms or nicknames. Researching the meaning of names may help narrow your search to find the perfect moniker for your new addition.

Perfect Pear of Jeans

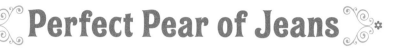

During pregnancy, your body will reconfigure itself so many times that even your new maternity jeans won't fit anymore. Stop sucking in your stomach and suck down a Perfect Pear of Jeans instead.

- **1 pear, cut into slices or cubes (reserve a slice for garnish)**
- **5 ounces lemon-lime soda**
- **1 teaspoon lime juice**

Place all the ingredients in a blender and pulse on medium-high speed just until the pear is pureed and the drink has a frothy consistency. Garnish with a slice of fresh pear and enjoy!

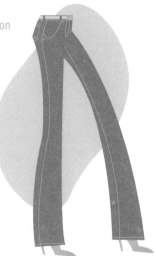

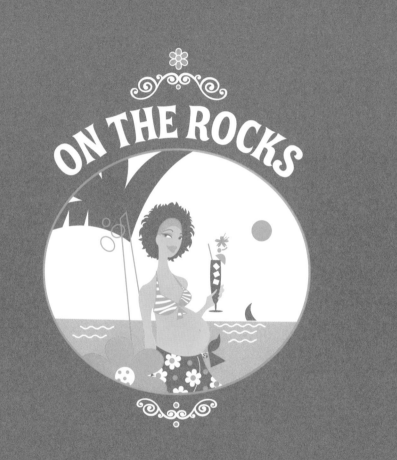

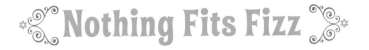

Nothing Fits Fizz

Your pants are getting tight, but rather than looking pregnant, you just look like you ate too much for lunch! Find a pair of elastic sweats and slide into a lounge chair with a refreshing Nothing Fits Fizz. It'll ease the frustration of growing out of your favorite outfits.

- **8 to 10 mint leaves**
- **4 ounces mango juice**
- **4 ounces club soda**
- **2 lime wedges**

In the bottom of a tall glass, muddle the mint leaves with the mango juice. Add ice, then fill the glass with club soda. Squeeze one lime wedge into the glass and garnish with the other.

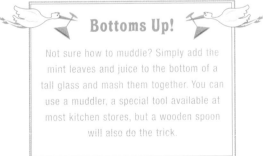

Bottoms Up!

Not sure how to muddle? Simply add the mint leaves and juice to the bottom of a tall glass and mash them together. You can use a muddler, a special tool available at most kitchen stores, but a wooden spoon will also do the trick.

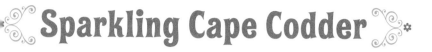

Sparkling Cape Codder

If you can't get to that New England beach this summer, a Sparkling Cape Codder is the next best thing. Take a sip, close your eyes, and imagine introducing your little one to the crisp Atlantic Ocean.

- **5 ounces cranberry juice**
- **4 ounces ginger ale**

Fill a tall glass with ice. Add all the ingredients and stir.

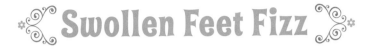

Swollen Feet Fizz

Once your favorite fashion accessory, now just a dreaded requirement. Kick off those too-tight mules and sit back with a Swollen Feet Fizz. The extra liquid may help rid your body of impurities and make the swelling subside.

- **2 ounces apple juice**
- **5 ounces sparkling water**
- **2 ounces cranberry juice**

Fill a tall glass with ice. Add all the ingredients and stir.

Bottoms Up!

Are your feet growing, along with your belly? Fluids increase during pregnancy and hormones slow circulation, so soon enough everything gives in to gravity and settles—you guessed it— in your feet, hands, and ankles. A few simple recommendations: Wear comfortable shoes, avoid prolonged standing, elevate your feet for an hour, increase fluid intake, and avoid salt.

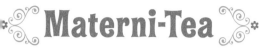 Materni-Tea

If you belong to a group of expectant mothers, have them over for an afternoon Materni-Tea and crustless finger sandwiches. You'll all feel elegant in spite of your ever-growing bumps.

- **5 ounces decaffeinated iced tea**
- **4 ounces cranberry juice**

Mix the tea and cranberry juice together in a tall glass and serve over ice.

A Toast to Your Health!

The jury is out on drinking herbal teas during pregnancy. Professionals disagree about the safety of many herbs, and the effects they may have on a developing fetus are not fully studied. The best advice is to consume them in moderation and to select only those teas that contain known nontoxic herbs. The U.S. Food and Drug Administration publishes a list of herbs approved for food use, and these are generally considered safe for beverages as well.

Doctor's Orders

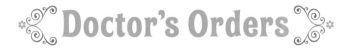

You've heard it time and again: Avoid stress! Heed your physician's advice. Fill a tall glass with Doctor's Orders and take it easy.

- **5 ounces lemon-lime soda**
- **3 ounces pineapple juice**
- **1 teaspoon grenadine**
- **Maraschino cherries, for garnish**
- **Fresh pineapple slice, for garnish**

Fill a tall glass with ice. Add all the ingredients and stir. Garnish with maraschino cherries and a slice of fresh pineapple and serve.

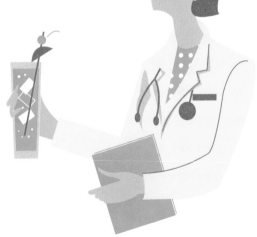

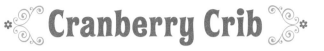

Cranberry Crib

When the weight of pregnancy is slowing you down and the crib you painstakingly built looks a little too inviting, wake up your senses with a tart, sparkling Cranberry Crib.

- 3 ounces cranberry juice
- 1 ounce orange juice
- 4 ounces plain seltzer
- Orange slice, for garnish

Fill a tall glass with ice. Add all the ingredients and stir. Garnish with an orange slice.

Basil Pomegranate Lemonade

This unique and exciting beverage is perfect for impressing your pregnant girl-friends at parties. The sophisticated flavors of pomegranate and basil combine with the familiar citrus to create a surprising and delightful thirst-quencher.

- **6 to 8 basil leaves**
- **2 ounces pomegranate juice**
- **4 ounces lemonade**
- **2 ounces lemon-lime soda**

Muddle basil and pomegranate juice in the bottom of a tall glass. Fill the glass with ice, add the lemonade and lemon-lime soda, and stir.

A Toast to Your Health!

Recent studies show that expectant moms who consume pomegranate juice may help reduce the risk of hypoxia ischemia, or decreased blood flow and oxygen to the brain, in infants born prematurely. Pomegranates contain high concentrations of polyphenols, substances that some scientists believe offer potential protective benefits to the nervous system.

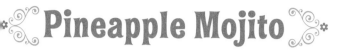

Pineapple Mojito

Drink a cool Pineapple Mojito as you pack your bag for a quick getaway to the hospital. Its tropical flavors will trick you into thinking you're getting ready for an island vacation. You'll be hula dancing all the way to the delivery room!

- **8 to 10 fresh mint leaves**
- **Juice from 1/2 lime**
- **1 teaspoon sugar**
- **3 ounces pineapple juice**
- **4 ounces club soda**
- **Lime slice, for garnish**

In the bottom of a tall glass, muddle the mint leaves with the lime juice and sugar. Add the pineapple juice, then fill the glass with ice and top off with club soda. Stir together with a straw and garnish with a slice of lime.

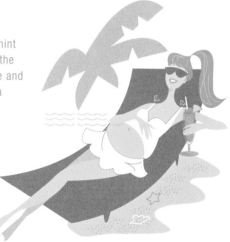

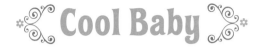

Cool Baby

The Cool Baby is a simple pleasure that's the perfect pick-me-up after you've been shopping all day to furnish the nursery for your new housemate.

- **4 ounces pineapple juice**
- **5 ounces club soda**
- **Fresh pineapple wedge (for garnish)**
- **Maraschino cherry (for garnish)**

Mix the pineapple juice and club soda together in a tall glass over ice. Garnish with a fresh pineapple wedge and a maraschino cherry and serve.

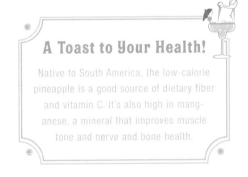

A Toast to Your Health!

Native to South America, the low-calorie pineapple is a good source of dietary fiber and vitamin C. It's also high in manganese, a mineral that improves muscle tone and nerve and bone health.

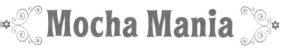

Mocha Mania

A fast, easy Mocha Mania is a perfect coffee-flavored concoction you can make in your own kitchen, allowing you to bypass the long line at the coffee shop entirely.

- **4 ounces decaffeinated iced coffee**
- **4 ounces chocolate milk**

Fill a tall glass with ice. Add coffee and chocolate milk. Mix with a straw and enjoy!

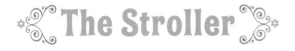

The Stroller

Choosing the right stroller can be overwhelming, especially when you're faced with deciphering all the high-tech features and complex folding mechanisms. If it all seems just too much, take this simple drink for a spin before you lose your cool.

- **6 ounces limeade**
- **8 to 10 fresh basil leaves**

Muddle the basil leaves with 2 ounces of limeade in the bottom of a tall glass. Add ice, fill with the rest of the limeade, and serve.

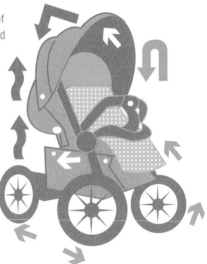

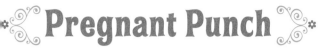

Pregnant Punch

When you're feeling your bloated, hormonal worst, it's tempting to take it out on your partner. But before you haul off and punch him, mix yourself a tall, cool Pregnant Punch. It's better for both of you. Honest.

- 1 ounce cranberry juice
- 1 ounce pineapple juice
- 2 ounces grapefruit juice
- 4 ounces ginger ale
- Pineapple wedge, for garnish

Fill a tall glass with ice. Add all the ingredients, stir, and garnish with a fresh pineapple wedge. Take a deep breath, relax, and enjoy.

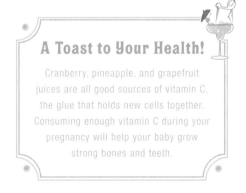

A Toast to Your Health!

Cranberry, pineapple, and grapefruit juices are all good sources of vitamin C, the glue that holds new cells together. Consuming enough vitamin C during your pregnancy will help your baby grow strong bones and teeth.

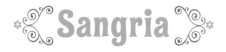

Sangria

Does pregnancy have you craving a great Spanish feast? Complement your tasty tapas with a refreshing pitcher of this fantastic Sangria. Raise your glass and say olé!

- **6 ounces white grape juice**
- **4 ounces purple grape juice**
- **4 ounces peach juice**
- **5 ounces pineapple juice**
- **1 tablespoon lime juice**
- **2 ounces orange juice**
- **1 tablespoon lemon juice**
- **Fresh lemon wedges, for serving**
- **Fresh peach wedges, for serving**

Mix all the ingredients together and refrigerate for at least 4 hours. Serve with fresh lemon and peach wedges. Makes 2 to 3 servings.

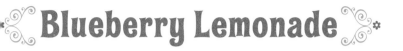

Blueberry Lemonade

Here's a flavorful blend that puts a colorful twist on the usual lemonade. Indulge in a glass when you're looking for decorating inspiration. You may be tempted to experiment with an entirely new hue!

- **3 ounces blueberry juice**
- **5 ounces lemonade**
- **Fresh blueberries, for garnish**

Fill a tall glass with ice. Add the blueberry juice, fill with lemonade, and stir. Garnish with fresh blueberries.

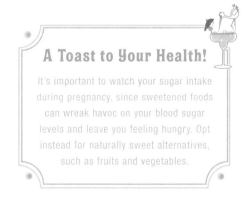

A Toast to Your Health!

It's important to watch your sugar intake during pregnancy, since sweetened foods can wreak havoc on your blood sugar levels and leave you feeling hungry. Opt instead for naturally sweet alternatives, such as fruits and vegetables.

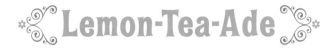

Lemon-Tea-Ade

When the sun is broiling hot and your pregnant body needs to cool down fast, Lemon-Tea-Ade is the ideal drink for instant refreshment. Pour. Stir. Drink. Ahhhhh!

- **6 ounces decaffeinated iced tea**
- **6 ounces lemonade**
- **Lemon wedge, for garnish**

Fill a tall glass with ice. Add all the ingredients and stir. Garnish with a lemon wedge.

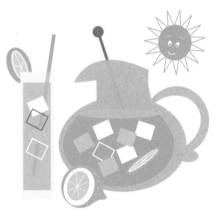

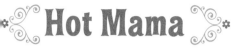

Hot Mama

You're such a good girl. You keep your emotions under control—at least when you're in public. You even smile at your in-laws! Show your true colors with a fiery Hot Mama, a spicy drink with all the flavor of a Bloody Mary but with ingredients appropriate for moms-to-be.

- 6 ounces tomato juice
- 1 teaspoon lemon juice
- 1/2 teaspoon Worcestershire sauce
- 3 drops hot sauce
- Lime wedge
- Freshly ground black pepper
- Celery stick (optional)

In a tall glass, mix together the tomato juice, lemon juice, Worcestershire sauce, and hot sauce. Squeeze in a lime wedge. Add pepper to taste. Serve over ice, garnished with a celery stick.

Bottoms Up!

Spicy foods—to eat or not to eat? According to researchers, strong-flavored foods do not seem to affect a fetus negatively or positively. Many cultures worldwide enjoy spicy cuisine with no known ill (or positive) effects. But such foods are best avoided if they give you heartburn or other discomfort.

Bouncing Baby

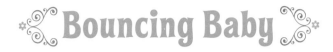

How many times have people asked you if you can feel the baby kick? Do they ask to feel your stomach? Before you haul off and bounce someone's head off the wall, calm yourself with a Bouncing Baby, an easy treat to mix and savor.

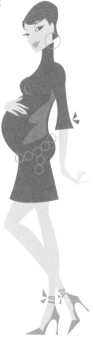

- **5 ounces fruit punch**
- **3 ounces fruit-flavored seltzer**
- **Orange slice, for garnish**

Fill a tall glass with ice. Add all the ingredients and stir. Garnish with an orange slice.

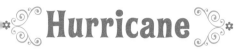

Hurricane

When you feel like you're spinning in circles, trying to get everything done before the big day, let the wind fill your sails with the rich flavors of a Hurricane, one of the South's most famous drinks.

- **2 ounces pineapple juice**
- **2 ounces passion-fruit juice**
- **1½ ounces lemonade**
- **1 ounce orange juice**
- **2 tablespoons lime juice**
- **½ teaspoon grenadine**

Fill a cocktail shaker with ice. Add all the ingredients and shake well. Strain into a martini glass and serve.

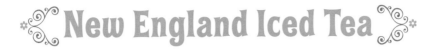

New England Iced Tea

If you like iced tea like I do, then anytime is teatime. You'll love the light yet interesting flavor of the New England Iced Tea!

- **4 ounces blueberry juice**
- **4 ounces decaffeinated iced tea**
- **Fresh blueberries, for garnish**

Fill a tall glass with ice. Add all the ingredients and stir. Garnish with fresh blueberries.

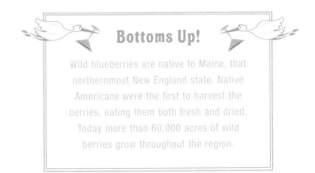

Bottoms Up!

Wild blueberries are native to Maine, that northernmost New England state. Native Americans were the first to harvest the berries, eating them both fresh and dried. Today more than 60,000 acres of wild berries grow throughout the region.

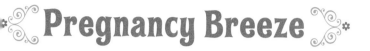

Pregnancy Breeze

Walking around with extra pounds is no easy task. But the Pregnancy Breeze is a flavorful combination that will be a breeze for you, anytime.

- **3 ounces cranberry juice**
- **4 ounces grapefruit juice**
- **2 teaspoons grenadine**

Fill a tall glass with ice. Add all the ingredients, stir, and serve.

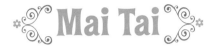
Mai Tai

Your honeymoon seems like an eternity ago. Where once you were browsing beautiful resort brochures, now you're flipping through baby-name books and toy catalogs. Step back in time and enjoy a Mai Tai! The flavors will remind you of good times past, even as you look forward to the fun of future vacations at child-friendly family resorts.

- **4 ounces pineapple juice**
- **2 ounces club soda**
- **1 teaspoon grenadine**
- **4 ounces orange juice**
- **1 tablespoon cream of coconut**

Fill a tall glass with ice. Add all the ingredients, stir, and serve.

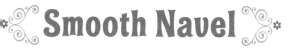

Smooth Navel

Remember those days when you could see your toes without your belly button blocking your view? Indulge yourself with a Smooth Navel, a sweet elixir that will even out the tensions of the day.

- 2 ounces peach juice
- 5 ounces fresh-squeezed orange juice
- Peach slice, for garnish

Fill a tall glass with ice. Add the juices and stir. Garnish with a fresh peach slice.

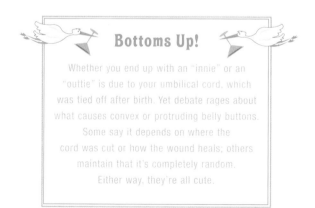

Bottoms Up!

Whether you end up with an "innie" or an "outtie" is due to your umbilical cord, which was tied off after birth. Yet debate rages about what causes convex or protruding belly buttons. Some say it depends on where the cord was cut or how the wound heals; others maintain that it's completely random. Either way, they're all cute.

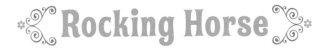

Rocking Horse

When the extra pounds add up and you feel more like you should be let out to pasture than sipping drinks with the glamorous crowd at the Kentucky Derby, mix up a Rocking Horse. You'll immediately be transformed into a sociable Southern belle.

- **8 to 10 fresh mint leaves**
- **1 teaspoon lemon juice**
- **1 teaspoon sugar**
- **6 ounces ginger ale**

In the bottom of a tall glass, muddle mint leaves with lemon juice. Add ice, sugar, and ginger ale and stir. Serve with a straw.

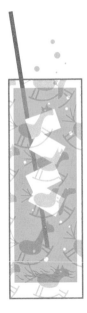

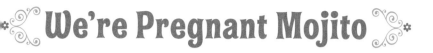

We're Pregnant Mojito

One of the greatest joys of pregnancy is telling your family and friends that you're going to have a baby. The pleasant flavor of the muddled cucumber, accented with an unexpected hint of basil, makes the We're Pregnant Mojito the perfect drink for toasting your exciting news.

- **¼ cup peeled cucumber, diced**
- **1 teaspoon lime juice**
- **4 to 5 fresh basil leaves**
- **5 ounces ginger ale**

In the bottom of a tall glass, muddle the cucumber, lime juice, and basil. Fill a glass with ice. Add ginger ale, stir, and serve.

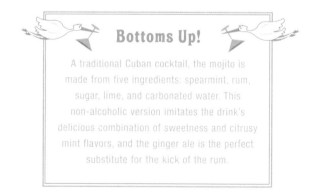

Bottoms Up!

A traditional Cuban cocktail, the mojito is made from five ingredients: spearmint, rum, sugar, lime, and carbonated water. This non-alcoholic version imitates the drink's delicious combination of sweetness and citrusy mint flavors, and the ginger ale is the perfect substitute for the kick of the rum.

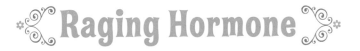

Raging Hormone

Do you cry while watching your favorite cooking show? Do you yell at your partner because the house is a mess? Seek emotional balance with a Raging Hormone, a great excuse for you to take a load off and relax.

- **6 to 7 mint leaves**
- **1 ounce lemonade**
- **2 ounces cherry juice**
- **4 ounces ginger ale**

In the bottom of a tall glass, muddle mint leaves, lemonade, and cherry juice. Add ice and ginger ale. Stir and serve immediately.

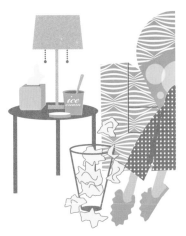

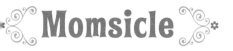 Momsicle

You've heard of the Popsicle. Now try the Momsicle! The fruit juices and sparkling water will provide the same fun, minus the fudgy calories.

- **2 ounces pineapple juice**
- **2 ounces pear juice**
- **1 ounce blueberry juice**
- **1 teaspoon lime juice**
- **2 ounces sparkling water**

Fill a tall glass with ice. Add all the ingredients, stir, and serve.

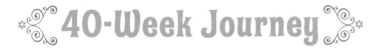

40-Week Journey

Being pregnant has its ups and downs, but in the end you can look back on an amazing period of growth, both physical and emotional. Commemorate your evolution with a 40-Week Journey. It tastes so good, you just might want to be a repeat traveler.

- **2 ounces fresh-squeezed orange juice**
- **5 ounces vanilla seltzer**
- **Orange slice, for garnish**

Pour the orange juice and seltzer into a tall glass. Fill the glass with ice and stir. Garnish with a fresh orange slice.

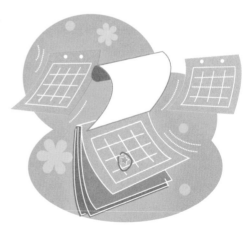

Preemie Punch

Good things come in small packages. Mix together this Preemie Punch and remember to enjoy every day with your future little one. They get big fast!

- 3 ounces pineapple juice
- 2 ounces cranberry juice
- 2 ounces lemon-lime soda
- ½ teaspoon grenadine
- Fresh pineapple wedge (for garnish)

Mix all ingredients in a tall glass over ice. Garnish with a fresh pineapple wedge and serve.

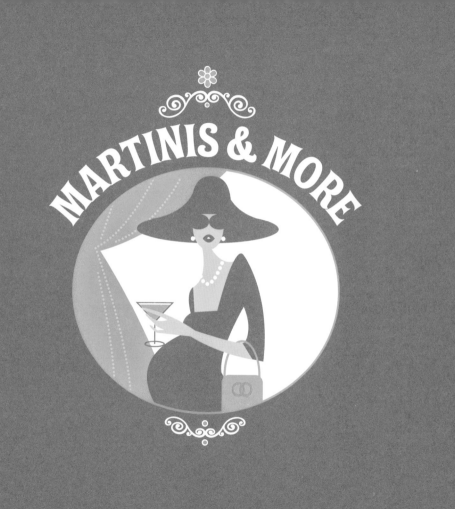

MARTINIS & MORE

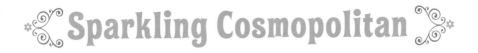

Sparkling Cosmopolitan

When I first became pregnant, I wondered how I'd live without a Cosmo, that cranberry-flavored cocktail. I created the Sparkling Cosmopolitan so I wouldn't have to. With this magical elixir in your favorite martini glass, you'll never miss the real thing.

- **3 ounces cranberry juice**
- **5 ounces orange-flavored sparkling water**
- **1 lime wedge**

Mix together the juice and sparkling water, then squeeze in the lime. Serve straight up in a martini glass.

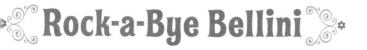

Rock-a-Bye Bellini

If your morning sickness feels more like all-day sickness, soothe your nausea with a Rock-a-Bye Bellini. The ginger ale will help settle your stomach, and the peaches will give you energy.

- **4 to 5 frozen peach slices**
- **5 ounces ginger ale**

Puree the peaches in a blender, then stir in the ginger ale. If you're feeling fancy, serve the drink in a champagne flute.

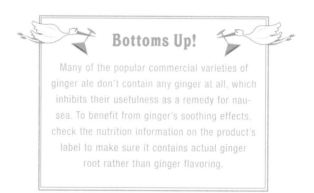

Bottoms Up!

Many of the popular commercial varieties of ginger ale don't contain any ginger at all, which inhibits their usefulness as a remedy for nausea. To benefit from ginger's soothing effects, check the nutrition information on the product's label to make sure it contains actual ginger root rather than ginger flavoring.

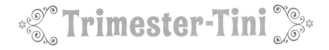

Trimester-Tini

Your calendar becomes your best friend as you track your progress through this nine-month adventure. Celebrate each benchmark with the Trimester-Tini, a fresh-fruit beverage you'll want to share with friends.

- **10 to 15 fresh blueberries**
- **1 teaspoon lime juice**
- **5 ounces ginger ale**

Muddle the blueberries in a martini glass. Mix the lime juice, ginger ale, and ice in a cocktail shaker. Shake well and strain into the martini glass.

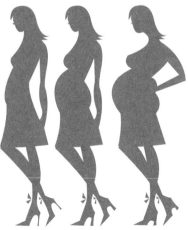

Easy Delivery

Creating a birth plan is a good way to ensure an easy (or, at least, an easier) delivery. So write down your wishes and directions for how you'd like the big day to go. Then review them with your partner over the liquid version of your Easy Delivery.

- 2 ounces peach juice
- ½ teaspoon sugar
- ½ teaspoon lemon juice
- 3 ounces ginger ale
- ½ cup ice

Shake together all the ingredients in a cocktail shaker. Strain into a chilled martini glass and serve immediately.

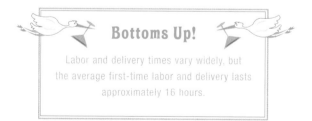

Bottoms Up!

Labor and delivery times vary widely, but the average first-time labor and delivery lasts approximately 16 hours.

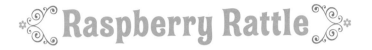

Raspberry Rattle

Every once in a while, it's easy to get rattled with all the errands you need to run, the doctors you need to see, and the questions you have to answer. When all your new responsibilities are getting to you, chill out with a sparkling Raspberry Rattle.

- **4 ounces raspberry-flavored sparkling water**
- **3 ounces raspberry juice**
- **8 to 10 frozen raspberries**
- **1 teaspoon grenadine**

Mix together all the ingredients in a cocktail shaker. Serve straight up in a martini glass.

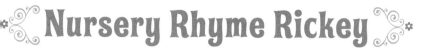

Nursery Rhyme Rickey

The lime-fresh Nursery Rhyme Rickey is sure to be a classic in your drink repertoire.

- **4 ounces lemon lime soda**
- **Juice of ½ lime**
- **1 ounce grenadine**

Mix together all the ingredients in a cocktail shaker. Serve straight up in a martini glass.

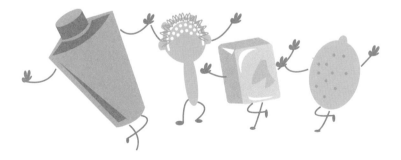

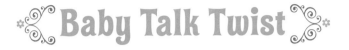

Baby Talk Twist

I have a full library of baby "progress" books: what to expect when baby is so many weeks, months, years. As all the expectations begin to build, suck down a Baby Talk Twist and remember that each and every baby sparkles with individuality.

- **4 ounces orange-flavored seltzer**
- **1 ounce orange juice**
- **1 ounce grenadine**

Mix together all the ingredients in a cocktail shaker. Serve straight up in a martini glass.

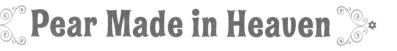

Pear Made in Heaven

Having twins? Whether they're two of a kind or one of each flavor, celebrate your excitement with a Pear Made in Heaven.

- **Sugar for rim of glass**
- **Lemon wedge**
- **2 ounces pear juice**
- **3 ounces ginger ale**
- **½ teaspoon honey**
- **1 ounce blueberry juice**

Fill a shallow plate with sugar. Wipe the edge of a martini glass with a lemon wedge. Dip the glass in the sugar to coat. Pour the pear juice, ginger ale, honey, and blueberry juice into a cocktail shaker, add some ice, shake, and strain. Serve straight up in the sugar-rimmed glass.

Bottoms Up!

What are the chances you'll give birth to twins (or triplets or more)? According to recent statistics, they could be as great as 1 in 33. Factors that may increase the chances are a family history of multiple births, use of fertility drugs, or race. Women who conceive at age 30 or older also enjoy increased odds.

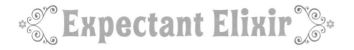

Expectant Elixir

Looking for something warm and comforting to ease your mind on chilly days? Try the Expectant Elixir, a perfect blend for chasing away your worries.

- **8 ounces hot herbal tea**
- **4 to 5 fresh mint leaves**
- **1 tablespoon honey**

Brew a fresh pot of tea. Pour into mug, then stir in mint and honey. Sip immediately.

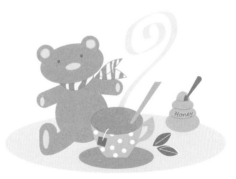

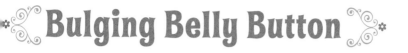

Bulging Belly Button

It's a tattoo! It's a beauty mark! No, it's a bulging belly button! There's no need for plastic surgery—make yourself a Bulging Belly Button to remind yourself that your newfound protrusion should disappear with the arrival of your baby.

- **1 teaspoon coffee syrup**
- **2 ounces raspberry juice**
- **2 ounces white grape juice**
- **1 teaspoon chocolate syrup, for garnish**

Mix together all the ingredients in a martini glass. Serve straight up, drizzled with chocolate syrup.

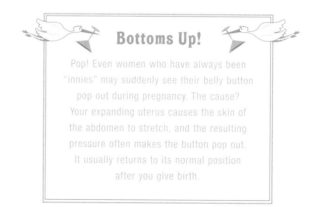

Bottoms Up!

Pop! Even women who have always been "innies" may suddenly see their belly button pop out during pregnancy. The cause? Your expanding uterus causes the skin of the abdomen to stretch, and the resulting pressure often makes the button pop out. It usually returns to its normal position after you give birth.

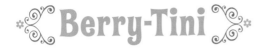

Berry-Tini

Break up the monotony of your day with the exotic flavor of fresh blackberries. A Berry-Tini will turn the ordinary into the extraordinary.

- **8 fresh blackberries**
- **5 ounces lemon-lime soda**
- **1/2 teaspoon fresh lime juice**

Muddle blackberries in a cocktail shaker. Add soda, lime juice, and ice. Shake well, then strain into a martini glass and serve.

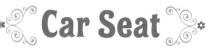

Car Seat

Installing a car seat can take hours and may prove to be a stressful experience. Pair up with your partner: One reads the directions while the other attempts to follow them. After you've finished the project, relax in your own easy chair with a citrusy Car Seat.

- **2 ounces fresh-squeezed blood orange juice**
- **3 ounces ginger ale**
- **1 teaspoon lime juice**

Mix together all the ingredients in a cocktail shaker. Strain into a martini glass and serve.

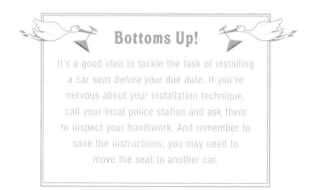

Bottoms Up!

It's a good idea to tackle the task of installing a car seat *before* your due date. If you're nervous about your installation technique, call your local police station and ask them to inspect your handiwork. And remember to save the instructions; you may need to move the seat to another car.

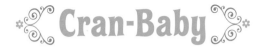

Cran-Baby

Cool autumn days call for heartwarming beverages. Make your entire body feel good with the Cran-Baby's blend of homey apple, cinnamon, and nutmeg flavors, with a special twist of cranberry to mix things up a little.

- **5 ounces pasteurized apple cider**
- **2 ounces cranberry juice**
- **Cinnamon stick**
- **Dash of nutmeg, for garnish**

Heat all the ingredients in a small saucepan, stirring until warm. Pour into a mug, sprinkle on a dash of nutmeg, and serve immediately.

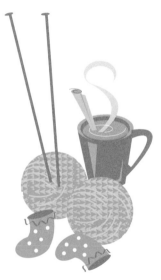

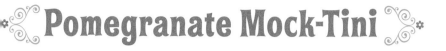

Pomegranate Mock-Tini

Don't miss out on the holiday fun. Grab a martini glass off the shelf and join in the party! The Pomegranate Mock-Tini is the perfect holiday drink—it's simple to make and will keep you from envying your cocktail-sipping friends.

- **2 ounces pomegranate juice**
- **4 ounces lemon-lime soda**

Stir all the ingredients together. Serve straight up in a martini glass.

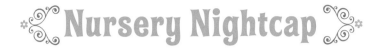

Nursery Nightcap

At the end of a busy day, wind down with a soothing Nursery Nightcap. The herbal tea will help you relax, and the shot of vanilla syrup will be a sweet treat to inspire happy dreams.

- **8 ounces hot herbal decaffeinated tea**
- **½ teaspoon vanilla syrup**

Brew hot decaffeinated tea. Add vanilla syrup and stir. Enjoy immediately.

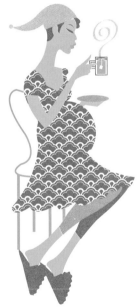

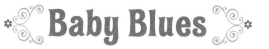

Baby Blues

Don't let pregnancy get you down! Pick yourself up with a Baby Blues mocktail. The vanilla syrup, crushed graham cracker, cinnamon, and sugar are a great combo for lifting your spirits and making pregnancy a fun, sweet time!

- 1 graham cracker
- Lime wedge
- 2 ounces vanilla seltzer
- 2 ounces ginger ale
- 1 ounce blueberry juice
- Pinch of cinnamon, for garnish

Place a graham cracker in a baggie and use your fingers to crumble it. Place crumbs in a small dish. Wipe the edge of a martini glass with a lime wedge, then dip the glass on the plate to coat the rim with crumbs.

In a cocktail shaker, mix vanilla seltzer, ginger ale, blueberry juice, and ice. Strain into the martini glass and add a pinch of cinnamon on top!

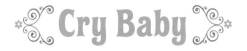
Cry Baby

As you've probably experienced, hormones can make you weepy just about anywhere, anytime. Next time the tears come, make yourself a Cry Baby—the cherry on top will help make it all better!

- **1½ teaspoons grenadine**
- **1 tablespoon cherry juice**
- **4 ounces vanilla seltzer**
- **½ cup ice**
- **Maraschino cherry, for garnish**

Shake together all the ingredients in a cocktail shaker. Strain into a martini glass and garnish with a maraschino cherry.

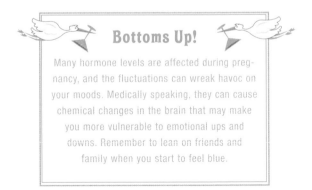

Bottoms Up!

Many hormone levels are affected during pregnancy, and the fluctuations can wreak havoc on your moods. Medically speaking, they can cause chemical changes in the brain that may make you more vulnerable to emotional ups and downs. Remember to lean on friends and family when you start to feel blue.

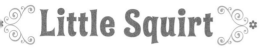

Little Squirt

Pucker up with a Little Squirt, an energizing pick-me-up that packs a punch with its lemony tartness.

- **Sugar for rim of glass**
- **Lemon wedge**
- **5 ounces lemon-lime soda**
- **1 tablespoon fresh lemon juice**

Fill a shallow plate with sugar. Wipe the edge of a martini glass with a lemon wedge. Dip the glass in the sugar to coat the rim.

In a cocktail shaker, mix the lemon-lime soda and lemon juice. Shake well and strain into the martini glass.

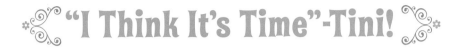

"I Think It's Time"-Tini!

Whether your baby's due in January or July, anytime's the right time for the "I Think It's Time"–Tini. The tropical blend of coconut, mango, and pineapple juices will warm you with thoughts of summer in midwinter and will quench your thirst in midsummer.

- **3 ounces ginger ale**
- **1 ounce mango juice**
- **1 ounce pineapple juice**
- **Coconut shavings, for garnish**

In a cocktail shaker, mix the ginger ale, mango juice, and pineapple juice. Shake well and strain into a martini glass. Add a pinch of coconut shavings on top.

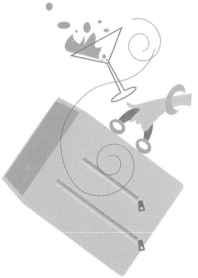

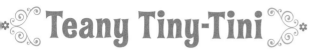

Teany Tiny-Tini

A little tea mixed with your pregnancy-safe martini makes this teatime the best time!

- 3 ounces decaffeinated iced tea
- 2 ounces ginger ale
- 1 teaspoon honey
- ¼ teaspoon lemon juice

Mix together all the ingredients. Serve straight up in a martini glass.

Basil Mock-Tini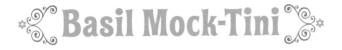

Enjoy the unique, clean taste of the Basil Mock-Tini when you're out on the town. The fresh ingredients of this signature drink assure you of a fresh taste every time.

- **6 to 8 basil leaves**
- **1 ounce lime juice**
- **5 ounces club soda**
- **3 teaspoons sugar**

Muddle basil and lime juice in the bottom of a high-sided glass. Add the club soda and sugar, stir, and serve straight up in a martini glass.

A Toast to Your Health!

Basil is good for more than just a tasty pesto. It is believed to improve blood circulation during pregnancy and may even help combat morning sickness. Basil's strong taste may increase the production of saliva, aiding in digestion and helping to alleviate nausea.

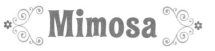

Mimosa

Tired of drinking decaffeinated coffee, plain orange juice, or water for breakfast? Try a Mimosa. It's a favorite breakfast drink that can be ready in a flash. There's no better way to start a beautiful new day.

- **2 ounces fresh-squeezed orange juice**
- **2 ounces ginger ale**

Fill a champagne glass halfway with orange juice. Add ginger ale and serve immediately.

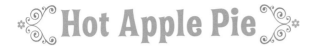

Hot Apple Pie

The Hot Apple Pie is the perfect accompaniment to a thick slice of cheddar cheese or a honey-dipped donut.

- **1 teaspoon vanilla syrup**
- **8 ounces pasteurized apple cider**
- **1 cinnamon stick**

Heat all the ingredients in a small saucepan, stirring until warm. Serve immediately in a mug.

A Toast to Your Health!

The perfect snack to fight fatigue: apples and cheese. Pairing complex carbohydrates with protein-dense foods may help you stay alert and cheerful throughout the day. And don't forget applesauce, which may help ease nausea—a good reason to keep a fresh jar in the fridge.

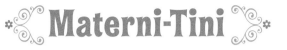

Materni-Tini

Holding a Materni-Tini will make you feel like you're in the height of style, even with a wardrobe full of oversized maternity clothes. Best of all, you can treat yourself to several cherries. Yum!

- **3 ounces orange juice**
- **1 ounce lime juice**
- **2 teaspoons grenadine**
- **Maraschino cherries, for garnish**

Mix all the ingredients together.
Serve straight up in a martini glass,
garnished with maraschino cherries.

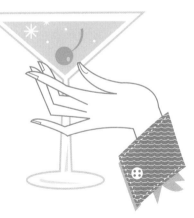

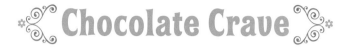

Chocolate Crave

Being pregnant provides the perfect excuse to enjoy a Chocolate Crave whenever you want!

- **4 ounces milk**
- **3 tablespoons chocolate syrup**
- **4 ounces seltzer**

Mix together the milk and chocolate syrup. Add the seltzer and serve immediately in a large glass.

A Toast to Your Health!

For many, pregnancy and cravings go hand in hand. But craving certain foods may not indicate that your body is lacking particular nutrients. The most common cravings are for red meat as well as tart, salty, and sweet foods. If you feel a craving coming on, take the opportunity to indulge in a healthy alternative. Remember to maintain a balanced diet and watch your caloric intake, too.

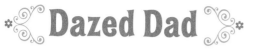

Dazed Dad

Whip up a Dazed Dad and relish the memory of the moment you told your honey about your delicate condition.

- 1 ounce orange juice
- 1 ounce pineapple juice
- 2 ounces lemon-lime soda
- ½ teaspoon grenadine
- Orange wedge, for garnish

Fill a cocktail shaker with ice. Add all the ingredients and shake well. Strain into a martini glass and garnish with an orange wedge.

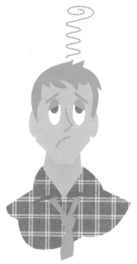

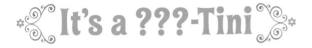

It's a ???-Tini

Life is full of surprises, and one of the best is the moment you find out if you're having a boy or a girl. Whether you decide to wait until the baby arrives or learn ahead of time, toast the excitement generated by the anticipation with an It's a ???-Tini.

- **2 ounces grape juice**
- **5 ounces pasteurized sparkling apple cider**

Combine all the ingredients in a martini glass. Serve straight up.

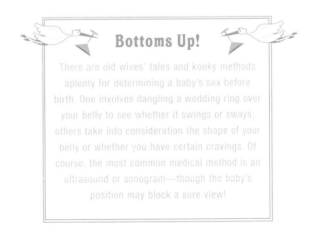

Bottoms Up!

There are old wives' tales and kooky methods aplenty for determining a baby's sex before birth. One involves dangling a wedding ring over your belly to see whether it swings or sways; others take into consideration the shape of your belly or whether you have certain cravings. Of course, the most common medical method is an ultrasound or sonogram—though the baby's position may block a sure view!

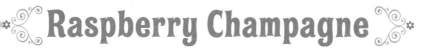

Raspberry Champagne

When you're out on the town with the girls but you're not quite ready to tell them your big news, order this drink at the bar to keep up appearances. To the casual observer, it will look like a real glass of Champagne. Your secret will be safe with the bartender!

- **4 to 6 fresh or frozen raspberries**
- **6 ounces pasteurized sparkling apple cider**

Place the raspberries in the bottom of a Champagne flute. Fill with the sparkling apple cider and serve immediately.

TABLE OF EQUIVALENCIES

U.S.	Metric
1/4 tsp	1.25 ml
1/2 tsp	2.5 ml
1 tsp	5 ml
1 tbsp (3 tsp)	15 ml
1 fl oz (2 tbsp)	30 ml
1/4 cup	60 ml
1/3 cup	80 ml
1/2 cup	120 ml
1 pint (2 cups)	480 ml
1 quart (2 pints)	960 ml
1 gallon (4 quarts)	3.84 l

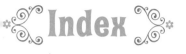

Index

ABOUT THE AUTHOR

Alyssa Dubin Gusenoff is the original nonalcoholic-drink guru. Originally from Piedmont, California, and now living in Newton, Massachusetts, Alyssa received her bachelor's degree in child development from Tufts University and a master's degree in speech pathology from Emerson College. When she's not mixing a tasty beverage for her husband, Dan, she's busy filling her son Zachary's sippy cup!

ACKNOWLEDGMENTS

Dan, long before Zack started kicking inside, you were pushing and kicking me to write down my ideas. You were my taste buds when all I could consume were oyster crackers and ginger ale. I can't thank you enough. I never would have finalized the recipes without you. I value your wit and your passion for success. I look forward to sharing many glasses of happiness with you.

Mom and Dad, you always supported my desire to write, from my elementary school attempts at a "Dubin Newsletter" to this book. You were always there to offer feedback. If only there were a way to make Piedmont and Newton closer.

Mom and Dad Gusenoff, your creativity is priceless. Thank you for helping to turn my black and white ideas into color. I couldn't write a better recipe for wonderful in-laws!

Thank you to Ed Claflin for sharing my excitement about this book from day one.

Many thanks to Melissa Wagner and everyone at Quirk Books. Your infectious enthusiasm for this project meant so much to me.

Thank you to all of the nurses and physicians in the NICU at Brigham and Women's Hospital, especially Dr. Marjorie Wilson, MaryAnne Bennett, Judy Panzeri-Hill, and Christine Kerble. Your stellar care gave me the peace of mind to go home at night and test the final recipes.

I raise my glass to all of my family and friends who were there for me during this adventure!